The Ketogenic Air Fryer Beginner's Cooking Guide

Tasty and Affordable Ketogenic Air Fryer Recipes to Start Your Day with the Right Foot

Nolan Turner

advice. The content within this book has been derived from various sources. Please consult a licensed professional before attempting any techniques outlined in this book.

By reading this document, the reader agrees that under no circumstances is the author responsible for any losses, direct or indirect, which are incurred as a result of the use of information contained within this document, including, but not limited to, — errors, omissions, or inaccuracies.

Table of Contents

Turmeric Zucchini Patties

Prep time: 15 minutes **Cooking time:** 10 minutes
Servings: 4

Ingredients:

2 zucchinis, trimmed, grated

1 egg yolk

½ teaspoon salt

1 teaspoon ground turmeric

½ teaspoon ground paprika

1 teaspoon cream cheese

3 tablespoons flax meal

1 teaspoon sesame oil

Directions:

Squeeze the juice from the zucchinis and put them in the big bowl. Add egg yolk, salt, ground turmeric, ground paprika, flax meal, and cream cheese. Stir the mixture well with the help of the spoon. Then make medium size patties from the zucchini mixture. Preheat the air fryer to

385F. Brush the air fryer basket with sesame oil and put the patties inside. Cook them for 5 minutes from each side.

Nutrition: calories 67, fat 4.7 fiber 2.8, carbs 5.5, protein 3.1

Herbed Asparagus and Sauce

Preparation time: 4 minutes **Cooking time:** 10 minutes **Servings**: 4

Ingredients:

1 pound asparagus, trimmed 2 tablespoons olive oil

A pinch of salt and black pepper 1 teaspoon garlic powder

1 teaspoon oregano, dried 1 cup Greek yogurt

cup basil, chopped

½ cup parsley, chopped

¼ cup chives, chopped

¼ cup lemon juice

garlic cloves, minced

Directions:

In a bowl, mix the asparagus with the oil, salt, pepper, oregano and garlic powder, and toss. Put the asparagus in the air fryer's basket and cook at 400 degrees F for 10 minutes. Meanwhile, in a blender, mix the yogurt with basil, chives, parsley, lemon juice and garlic cloves and pulse well. Divide the asparagus between plates, drizzle the sauce all over and serve.

Nutrition: calories 194, fat 6, fiber 2, carbs 4, protein8

Lemon Asparagus

Preparation time: 5 minutes **Cooking time:** 12 minutes **Servings**: 4

Ingredients:

1 pound asparagus, trimmed

A pinch of salt and black pepper 2 tablespoons olive oil

3 garlic cloves, minced

3 tablespoons parmesan, grated Juice of 1 lemon

Directions:

In a bowl, mix the asparagus with the rest of the ingredients and toss. Put the asparagus in your air fryer's basket and cook at 390 degrees F for 12 minutes. Divide between plates and serve.

Nutrition: calories 175, fat 5, fiber 2, carbs 4, protein8

Feta Peppers

Prep time: 15 minutes **Cooking time:** 10 minutes
Servings: 4

Ingredients:

5 oz Feta, crumbled

8 oz banana pepper, trimmed

1 teaspoon sesame oil

1 garlic clove, minced

½ teaspoon fresh dill, chopped

1 teaspoon lemon juice

½ teaspoon lime zest, grated

Directions:

Clean the seeds from the peppers and cut them into halves. Then sprinkle the peppers with sesame oil and put in the air fryer. Cook them for 10 minutes at 385F. Flip the peppers on another side after 5 minutes of cooking. Meanwhile, mix up minced garlic, fresh dill, lemon juice, and lime zest. Put the cooked banana peppers on the plate and sprinkle with lemon juice mixture. Then top the vegetables with crumbled feta.

Nutrition: calories 107, fat8.7, fiber 0.2, carbs 2.2, protein 5.2

Spicy Kale

Preparation time: 5 minutes **Cooking time:** 10 minutes **Servings**: 4

Ingredients:

1 pound kale, torn

1 tablespoon olive oil 1 teaspoon hot paprika

A pinch of salt and black pepper 2 tablespoons oregano, chopped

Directions:

In a pan that fits the air fryer, combine all the ingredients and toss. Put the pan in the air fryer and cook at 380 degrees F for 10 minutes. Divide between plates and serve.

Nutrition: calories 140, fat 3, fiber 2, carbs 3, protein 5

Buffalo Broccoli

Prep time: 15 minutes **Cooking time:** 6 minutes
Servings: 4

Ingredients:

2 cups broccoli florets

¼ cup of coconut milk

½ teaspoon salt

½ teaspoon chili flakes

1/3 cup coconut flour

1 tablespoon Buffalo sauce

Cooking spray

Directions:

Sprinkle the broccoli florets with salt and chili flakes. Then dip them in the coconut milk and coat in the coconut flour. Preheat the air fryer to 400F. Put the broccoli florets in the air fryer, spray with cooking spray, and cook them for 6 minutes. When the broccoli is cooked, transfer in the bowl and sprinkle with Buffalo sauce.

Nutrition: calories 98, fat 5.4, fiber 5.6, carbs 10.1, protein 3.6

Kale and Sprouts

Preparation time: 5 minutes **Cooking time:** 15 minutes **Servings**:8

Ingredients:

1 pound Brussels sprouts, trimmed 2 cups kale, torn

tablespoon olive oil

Salt and black pepper to the taste 3 ounces mozzarella, shredded

Directions:

In a pan that fits the air fryer, combine all the ingredients except the mozzarella and toss. Put the pan in the air fryer and cook at 380 degrees F for 15 minutes. Divide between plates, sprinkle the cheese on top and serve.

Nutrition: calories 170, fat 5, fiber 3, carbs 4, protein 7

Paprika Leeks

Prep time: 15 minutes **Cooking time:**8 minutes **Servings:** 3

Ingredients:

2 big leeks, roughly sliced

1 egg, beaten

½ teaspoon ground paprika

½ teaspoon salt

½ teaspoon ground turmeric

2 tablespoons almond flour

Cooking spray

Directions:

Sprinkle the leek slices with ground paprika, salt, and ground turmeric. After this, dip every leek slice in the egg and coat in the almond flour. Preheat the air fryer to 400f and put the leek bites inside. Spray them with the cooking spray and cook for8 minutes. Shake after 4 minutes of cooking.

Nutrition: calories 150, fat 10.9, fiber 3.3, carbs 9.2, protein 6.5

Coconut Broccoli

Preparation time: 5 minutes **Cooking time:** 30 minutes **Servings**: 4

Ingredients:

3 tablespoons ghee, melted 15 ounces coconut cream 2 eggs, whisked

2 cups cheddar, grated 1 cup parmesan, grated 1 tablespoon mustard

1 pound broccoli florets

A pinch of salt and black pepper 1 tablespoon parsley, chopped

Directions:

Grease a baking pan that fits the air fryer with the ghee and arrange the broccoli on the bottom. Add the cream, mustard, salt, pepper and the eggs and toss. Sprinkle the cheese on top, put the pan in the air fryer and cook at

380 degrees F for 30 minutes. Divide between plates and serve.

Nutrition: calories 244, fat 12, fiber 3, carbs 5, protein 12

Lemon Peppermint Bars

Prep time: 15 minutes **Cooking time:** 16 minutes
Servings: 8

Ingredients:

1 teaspoon peppermint

1 cup almond flour

1/3 cup peanut butter

½ teaspoon baking powder

1 teaspoon lemon juice

½ teaspoon orange zest, grated

Directions:

In the bowl, mix up almond flour, peppermint, baking powder, and orange zest. Then add peanut butter and lemon juice. Knead the non-sticky dough. Cut the dough on8 pieces and roll the balls. Press them gently to get the shape of the bars. Preheat the air fryer to 365F. Line the air fryer basket with baking paper. Put 4 cookies in the air fryer in one layer. Cook them for8 minutes. Remove the cooked bars from the air fryer. Repeat the same steps with uncooked bars.

Nutrition: calories84, fat 7.2, fiber 1.1, carbs 3.1, protein 3.5

Avocado Cream Pudding

Preparation time: 5 minutes **Cooking time:** 25 minutes Serving: 6

Ingredients:

4 small avocados, peeled, pitted and mashed 2 eggs, whisked

1 cup coconut milk

¾ cup swerve

teaspoon cinnamon powder

½ teaspoon ginger powder

Directions:

In a bowl, mix all the ingredients and whisk well. Pour into a pudding mould, put it in the air fryer and cook at 350 degrees F for 25 minutes. Serve warm.

Nutrition: calories 192, fat8, fiber 2, carbs 5, protein 4

Chocolate Candies

Prep time: 15 minutes **Cooking time:** 2 minutes
Servings: 4

Ingredients:

1 oz almonds, crushed

1 oz dark chocolate

2 tablespoons peanut butter

2 tablespoons heavy cream

Directions:

Preheat the air fryer to 390F. Chop the dark chocolate and put it in the air fryer mold. Add peanut butter and heavy cream. Stir the mixture and transfer in the air fryer. Cook it for 2 minutes or until it starts to be melt. Then line the air tray with parchment. Put the crushed almonds on the tray in one layer. Then pour the cooked chocolate mixture over the almonds.

Flatten gently if needed and let it cool. Crack the cooked chocolate layer into the candies.

Nutrition: calories 154, fat 12.9, fiber 1.9, carbs 7.4, protein 3.9

Berry Pudding

Preparation time: 5 minutes **Cooking time:** 15 minutes **Servings**: 6

Ingredients:

cups coconut cream 1/3 cup blackberries 1/3 cup blueberries

tablespoons swerve Zest of 1 lime, grated

Directions:

In a blender, combine all the ingredients and pulse well. Divide this into 6 small ramekins, put them in your air fryer and cook at 340 degrees F for 15 minutes. Serve cold.

Nutrition: calories 173, fat 3, fiber 1, carbs 4, protein 4

Butter Crumble

Prep time: 20 minutes **Cooking time:** 25 minutes
Servings: 4

Ingredients:

½ cup coconut flour

2 tablespoons butter, softened

2 tablespoon Erythritol

3 oz peanuts, crushed

1 tablespoon cream cheese

1 teaspoon baking powder

½ teaspoon lemon juice

Directions:

In the mixing bowl mix up coconut flour, butter, Erythritol, baking powder, and lemon juice. Stir the mixture until homogenous. Then place it in the freezer for 10 minutes. Meanwhile, mix up peanuts and cream cheese. Grate the frozen dough. Line the air fryer mold with baking paper. Then put ½ of grated dough in the mold and flatten it. Top it with cream cheese mixture. Then put remaining grated dough over the cream cheese mixture. Place the mold with the crumble in the air fryer and cook it for 25 minutes at 330F.

Nutrition: calories 252, fat 19.6, fiber 7.8, carbs 13.1, protein8.8

Stevia Cake

Preparation time: 5 minutes **Cooking time:** 40 minutes **Servings**: 6

Ingredients:

2 tablespoons ghee, melted 1 cup coconut, shredded

1 cup mashed avocado 3 tablespoons stevia

teaspoon cinamon powder

2 teaspoons cinnamon powder

Directions:

In a bowl, mix all the ingredients and stir well. Pour this into a cake pan lined with parchment paper, place the pan in the fryer and cook at 340 degrees F for 40 minutes. Cool the cake down, slice and serve.

Nutrition: calories 192, fat 4, fiber 2, carbs 5, protein 7

Sweet Balls

Prep time: 2 hours **Cooking time:** 5 minutes
Servings: 4

Ingredients:

1 tablespoon cream cheese

3 oz goat cheese

2 tablespoons almond flour

1 tablespoon coconut flour

1 egg, beaten

1 tablespoon Splenda

Cooking spray

Directions:

Mash the goat cheese and mix it up with cream cheese. Then add egg, Splenda, and almond flour. Stir the mixture until homogenous. Then make 4 balls and coat them in the coconut flour. Freeze the cheese balls for 2 hours. Preheat the air fryer to 390F. Then place the frozen balls in the air fryer, spray them with cooking spray and cook for 5 minutes or until the cheese balls are light brown.

Nutrition: calories 224, fat 16.8, fiber 2.3, carbs 7.7, protein 11.4

Chia Cinnamon Pudding

Preparation time: 10 minutes **Cooking time:** 25 minutes **Servings**: 6

Ingredients:

cups coconut cream 6 egg yolks, whisked 2 tablespoons stevia

¼ cup chia seeds

2 teaspoons cinnamon powder 1 tablespoon ghee, melted

Directions:

In a bowl, mix all the ingredients, whisk, divide into 6 ramekins, place them all in your air fryer and cook at 340 degrees F for 25 minutes. Cool the puddings down and serve.

Nutrition: calories 180, fat 4, fiber 2 carbs 5, protein 7

Seeds and Almond Cookies

Prep time: 15 minutes **Cooking time:** 9 minutes **Servings:** 6

Ingredients:

1 teaspoon chia seeds

1 teaspoon sesame seeds

1 tablespoon pumpkin seeds, crushed

1 egg, beaten

2 tablespoons Splenda

1 teaspoon vanilla extract

1 tablespoon butter

4 tablespoons almond flour

¼ teaspoon ground cloves

1 teaspoon avocado oil

Directions:

Put the chia seeds, sesame seeds, and pumpkin seeds in the bowl. Add egg, Splenda, vanilla extract, butter, avocado oil, and ground cloves. Then add almond flour and mix up the mixture until homogenous. Preheat the air fryer to 375F. Line the air fryer basket with baking paper. With the help of the scooper make the cookies and flatten them gently. Place the cookies in the air fryer. Arrange them in one layer. Cook the seeds cookies for 9 minutes.

Nutrition: calories 180, fat 13.7, fiber 3, carbs 9.6, protein 5.8

Cauliflower Rice Pudding

Preparation time: 5 minutes **Cooking time:** 25 minutes **Servings**: 4

Ingredients:

1 and ½ cups cauliflower rice 2 cups coconut milk

3 tablespoons stevia

2 tablespoons ghee, melted

4 plums, pitted and roughly chopped

Directions:

In a bowl, mix all the ingredients, toss, divide into ramekins, put them in the air fryer, and cook at 340 degrees F for 25 minutes. Cool down and serve.

Nutrition: calories 221, fat 4, fiber 1, carbs 3, protein 3

Cauliflower and Tomato Bake

Preparation time: 5 minutes **Cooking time:** 20 minutes **Servings**: 2

Ingredients:

1 cup heavy whipping cream 2 tablespoons basil pesto

Salt and black pepper to the taste Juice of ½ lemon

1 pound cauliflower, florets separated 4 ounces cherry tomatoes, halved

3 tablespoons ghee, melted

7 ounces cheddar cheese, grated

Directions:

Grease a baking pan that fits the air fryer with the ghee. Add the cauliflower, lemon juice, salt, pepper, the pesto and the cream and toss gently. Add the tomatoes, sprinkle the cheese on top, introduce the pan in the fryer and cook at 380 degrees F for 20 minutes. Divide between plates and serve as a side dish.

Nutrition: calories 200, fat 7, fiber 2, carbs 4, protein 7

Turmeric Tofu

Prep time: 10 minutes **Cooking time:** 9 minutes
Servings: 2

Ingredients:

6 oz tofu, cubed

1 teaspoon avocado oil

1 teaspoon apple cider vinegar

1 garlic clove, diced

¼ teaspoon ground turmeric

¼ teaspoon ground paprika

½ teaspoon dried cilantro

¼ teaspoon lemon zest, grated

Directions:

In the bowl mix up avocado oil, apple cider vinegar, diced garlic, ground turmeric, paprika, cilantro, and lime zest. Coat the tofu cubes in the oil mixture. Preheat the air fryer to 400F. Put the tofu cubes in the air fryer and cook them for 9 minutes. Shake the tofu cubes from time to time during cooking.

Nutrition: calories 67, fat 3.9, fiber 1.1, carbs 2.5, protein 7.2

Coconut Chives Sprouts

Preparation time: 5 minutes **Cooking time:** 20 minutes **Servings**: 4

Ingredients:

pound Brussels sprouts, trimmed and halved Salt and black pepper to the taste

tablespoons ghee, melted

½ cup coconut cream

2 tablespoons garlic, minced 1 tablespoon chives, chopped

Directions:

In your air fryer, mix the sprouts with the rest of the ingredients except the chives, toss well, introduce in the air fryer and cook them at 370 degrees F for 20 minutes. Divide the Brussels sprouts between plates, sprinkle the chives on top and serve as a side dish.

Nutrition: calories 194, fat 6, fiber 2, carbs 4, protein8

Cheesy Zucchini Tots

Prep time: 15 minutes **Cooking time:** 6 minutes
Servings: 4

Ingredients:

1 zucchini, grated

½ cup Mozzarella, shredded

1 egg, beaten

2 tablespoons almond flour

½ teaspoon ground black pepper

1 teaspoon coconut oil, melted

Directions:

Mix up grated zucchini, shredded Mozzarella, egg, almond flour, and ground black pepper. Then make the small zucchini tots with the help of the fingertips. Preheat the air fryer to 385F. Place the zucchini tots in the air fryer basket and cook for 3 minutes from each side or until the zucchini tots are golden brown.

Nutrition: calories 64, fat 4.7, fiber 1, carbs 2.8, protein 3.8

Creamy Broccoli and Cauliflower

Preparation time: 5 minutes **Cooking time:** 20 minutes **Servings**: 4

Ingredients:

15 ounces broccoli florets

10 ounces cauliflower florets 1 leek, chopped

2 spring onions, chopped

Salt and black pepper to the taste 2 ounces butter, melted

2 tablespoons mustard 1 cup sour cream

5 ounces mozzarella cheese, shredded

Directions:

In a baking pan that fits the air fryer, add the butter and spread it well. Add the broccoli, cauliflower and the rest of the ingredients except the mozzarella and toss. Sprinkle the cheese on top, introduce the pan in the air fryer and cook at 380 degrees F for 20 minutes. Divide between plates and serve as a side dish.

Nutrition: calories 242, fat 13, fiber 2, carbs 4, protein8

Mushroom Tots

Prep time: 15 minutes **Cooking time:** 6 minutes
Servings: 2

Ingredients:

1 cup white mushrooms, grinded

1 teaspoon onion powder

1 egg yolk

3 teaspoons flax meal

½ teaspoon ground black pepper

1 teaspoon avocado oil

1 tablespoon coconut flour

Directions:

Mix up grinded white mushrooms with onion powder, egg yolk, flax meal, ground black pepper, and coconut flour. When the mixture is smooth and homogenous, make the mushroom tots. Preheat the air fryer to 400F. Sprinkle the air fryer basket with melted coconut oil and put the mushroom tots inside. Cook them for 3 minutes. Then flip the mushroom tots on another side and cook them for 2-3 minutes more or until they are light brown.

Nutrition: calories 76, fat 4.6, fiber 3.2, carbs 6.2, protein 4.2

Chili Zucchini Balls

Prep time: 10 minutes **Cooking time:** 12 minutes **Servings:** 4

Ingredients:

¼ teaspoon salt

¼ teaspoon ground cumin

1 zucchini, grated

2 oz Provolone cheese, grated

¼ teaspoon chili flakes

1 egg, beaten

¼ cup coconut flour

1 teaspoon sunflower oil

Directions:

In the bowl mix up salt, ground cumin, zucchini, Provolone cheese, chili flakes, egg, and coconut flour. Stir the mass with the help of the spoon and make the small balls. Then line the air fryer basket with baking paper and sprinkle it with sunflower oil. Put the zucchini balls in the air fryer basket and cook them for 12 minutes at 375F. Shake the balls every 2 minutes to avoid burning.

Nutrition: calories 122, fat 7.4, fiber 3.7, carbs 7.3, protein 7.2

Buttery Cauliflower Mix

Preparation time: 5 minutes **Cooking time:** 15 minutes **Servings**: 4

Ingredients:

1 pound cauliflower florets, roughly grated 3 eggs, whisked

3 tablespoons butter, melted

Salt and black pepper to the taste 1 tablespoon sweet paprika

Directions:

Heat up a pan that fits the air fryer with the butter over high heat, add the cauliflower and brown for 5 minutes. Add whisked eggs, salt, pepper and the paprika, toss, introduce the pan in the fryer and cook at 400 degrees F for 10 minutes. Divide between plates and serve.

Nutrition: calories 153, fat 5, fiber 2, carbs 5, protein 5

Bacon Cabbage

Prep time: 5 minutes **Cooking time:** 12 minutes
Servings: 2

Ingredients:

8 oz Chinese cabbage, roughly chopped

2 oz bacon, chopped

1 tablespoon sunflower oil

½ teaspoon onion powder

½ teaspoon salt

Directions:

Cook the bacon at 400F for 10 minutes. Stir it from time to time. Then sprinkle it with onion powder and salt. Add Chinese cabbage and shake the mixture well. Cook it for 2 minutes. Then add sunflower oil, stir the meal and place in the serving plates.

Nutrition: calories 232, fat 19.1, fiber 1.2, carbs 3.4, protein 12.3

Zucchinis and Arugula Mix

Preparation time: 5 minutes **Cooking time:** 20 minutes **Servings**: 4

Ingredients:

1 pound zucchinis, sliced 1 tablespoon olive oil

Salt and white pepper to the taste 4 ounces arugula leaves

¼ cup chives, chopped 1 cup walnuts, chopped

Directions:

In a pan that fits the air fryer, combine all the ingredients except the arugula and walnuts, toss, put the pan in the machine and cook at 360 degrees F for 20 minutes. Transfer this to a salad bowl, add the arugula and the walnuts, toss and serve as a side salad.

Nutrition: calories 170, fat 4, fiber 1, carbs 4, protein 5

Sesame Lamb Chops

Prep time: 10 minutes **Cooking time:** 11 minutes **Servings:** 6

Ingredients:

6 lamb chops (3 oz each lamb chop)

1 tablespoon sesame oil

1 tablespoon za'atar seasonings

Directions:

Rub the lamb chops with za'atar seasonings and sprinkle with sesame oil. Preheat the air fryer to 400F. Then arrange the lamb chops in the air fryer in one layer and cook them for 5 minutes. Then flip the pork chops on another side and cook them for 6 minutes more.

Nutrition: calories 183, fat8.8, fiber 0.3, carbs 0.3, protein 24.2

Rosemary Steaks

Preparation time: 5 minutes **Cooking time:** 24 minutes **Servings**: 4

Ingredients:

4 rib eye steaks

A pinch of salt and black pepper 1 tablespoon olive oil

1 teaspoon sweet paprika 1 teaspoon cumin, ground

1 teaspoon resemary, chopped

Directions:

In a bowl, mix the steaks with the rest of the ingredients, toss and put them in your air fryer's basket. Cook at 380 degrees F for 12 minutes on each side, divide between plates and serve.

Nutrition: calories 283, fat 12, fiber 3, carbs 6, protein 17

Mustard Beef Mix

Prep time: 15 minutes **Cooking time:** 30 minutes
Servings: 7

Ingredients:

2-pound beef ribs, boneless

1 tablespoon Dijon mustard

1 tablespoon sunflower oil

1 teaspoon ground paprika

1 teaspoon cayenne pepper

Directions:

In the shallow bowl mix up Dijon mustard and sunflower oil. Then sprinkle the beef ribs with ground paprika and cayenne pepper. After this, brush the meat with Dijon mustard mixture and leave for 10 minutes to marinate. Meanwhile, preheat the air fryer to 400F. Put the beef ribs in the air fryer to and cook them for 10 minutes.

Then flip the ribs on another side and reduce the air fryer heat to 325F. Cook the ribs for 20 minutes more.

Nutrition: calories 262, fat 10.3, fiber 0.3, carbs 0.4, protein 39.5

Adobo Oregano Beef

Preparation time: 5 minutes **Cooking time:** 30 minutes **Servings:** 4

Ingredients:

pound beef roast, trimmed

½ teaspoon oregano, dried

¼ teaspoon garlic powder

A pinch of salt and black pepper

½ teaspoon turmeric powder 1 tablespoon olive oil

Directions:

In a bowl, mix the roast with the rest of the ingredients, and rub well. Put the roast in the air fryer's basket and cook at 390 degrees F for 30 minutes. Slice the roast, divide it between plates and serve with a side salad.

Nutrition: calories 294, fat 12, fiber 3, carbs 6, protein 19

Chili Loin Medallions

Prep time: 20 minutes **Cooking time:** 15 minutes
Servings: 4

Ingredients:

1-pound pork loin

4 oz bacon, sliced

1 teaspoon ground cumin

1 teaspoon coconut oil, melted

½ teaspoon salt

½ teaspoon chili flakes

Directions:

Slice the pork loin on the meat medallions and sprinkle them with ground cumin, salt, and chili flakes. Then wrap every meat medallion in the sliced bacon and sprinkle with coconut oil. Place the wrapped medallions in the air fryer basket in one layer and cook them for 10 minutes at 375F. Then carefully flip the meat medallions on another side and cook them for 5 minutes more.

Nutrition: calorie 440, fat 28.9, fiber 0.1, carbs 0.7, protein 41.6

Meatballs and Sauce

Preparation time: 5 minutes **Cooking time:** 25 minutes **Servings**: 4

Ingredients:

tablespoons olive oil

2 spring onions, chopped 1 egg, whisked

2 tablespoons rosemary, chopped 2 pounds beef, ground

1 garlic clove, minced

A pinch of salt and black pepper 24 ounces tomatoes, crushed

Directions:

In a bowl, mix the beef with all the ingredients except the oil and the tomatoes, stir well and shape medium meatballs out of this mix. Heat up a pan that fits the air fryer with the oil over medium-high heat, add the meatballs and cook for 2 minutes on each side. Add the tomatoes, toss, put the pan in the fryer and cook at 370 degrees F for 20 minutes. Divide into bowls and serve.

Nutrition: calories 273, fat 10, fiber 3, carbs 6, protein 15

Steak Rolls

Prep time: 25 minutes **Cooking time:** 18 minutes
Servings: 4

Ingredients:

12 oz pork steaks (3 oz each steak)

1 green bell pepper

2 oz asparagus, trimmed

1 teaspoon ground black pepper

¼ teaspoon salt

1 teaspoon sunflower oil

1 teaspoon chili flakes

1 teaspoon avocado oil

Directions:

Beat every pork steak with the kitchen hammer gently.
Then sprinkle the meat with chili flakes and avocado oil
and place it in the air fryer in one layer. Cook the meat

for8 minutes at 375F. Then remove the meat from the air fryer and cool to the room temperature. Meanwhile, cut the bell pepper on the thin wedges. Mix up together pepper wedges and asparagus. Add ground black pepper, salt, and sunflower oil. Mix up the vegetables. After this, place the vegetables on the pork steaks and roll them. Secure the meat with toothpicks if needed. Then transfer the steak bundles in the air fryer in one layer and cook them for 10 minutes at 365F.

Nutrition: calories 231, fat 13.3, fiber 0.9, carbs 3.2, protein 23.9

Basil Beef and Avocado

Preparation time: 5 minutes **Cooking time:** 25 minutes **Servings**: 4

Ingredients:

4 flank steaks

garlic clove, minced 1/3 cup beef stock

avocados, peeled, pitted and sliced 1 teaspoon chili flakes

½ cup basil, chopped

2 spring onions, chopped 2 teaspoons olive oil

A pinch of salt and black pepper

Directions:

Heat up a pan that fits the air fryer with the oil over medium-high heat, add the steaks and cook for 2 minutes on each side. Add the rest of the ingredients except the avocados, put the pan in the air fryer and cook at 380 degrees F for 15 minutes. Add the avocado slices, cook for 5 minutes more, divide everything between plates and serve.

Nutrition: calories 273, fat 12, fiber 3, carbs 6, protein 18

Nutmeg Baby Back Ribs

Prep time: 15 minutes **Cooking time:** 40 minutes
Servings: 3

Ingredients:

10 oz baby back ribs, roughly chopped

1 teaspoon ground cumin

½ teaspoon ground nutmeg

½ teaspoon salt

1 teaspoon cayenne pepper

1 tablespoon sunflower oil

1 teaspoon keto tomato sauce

1 tablespoon lemon juice

Directions:

In the mixing bowl mix up ground cumin, ground nutmeg, salt, cayenne pepper, sunflower oil, tomato sauce, lemon juice. Then rub the ribs with the spice mixture and leave for 10 minutes to marinate. Meanwhile, preheat the air fryer to 355F. Wrap the ribs in the foil and place it in the preheated air fryer. Cook the ribs for 40 minutes.

Nutrition: calories 262, fat 16.7, fiber 0.3, carbs 1.6, protein 25.1

Beef Casserole

Preparation time: 5 minutes **Cooking time:** 30 minutes **Servings**: 4

Ingredients:

1 tablespoon olive oil

1 and ½ cups coconut cream

½ cup parmesan, grated 1 pound beef, ground

1 bunch spring onions, chopped 1 tablespoon keto tomato sauce A pinch of salt and black pepper 2 cups cheddar cheese, ground

1 pound cherry tomatoes, chopped

Directions:

Heat up a pan with the oil over medium-high heat, add the beef and brown for 5 minutes. Add spring onions, tomatoes, salt and pepper and cook for 3-4 minutes more. Transfer this to a pan that fits the air fryer, pour the cream, sprinkle the parmesan and cheddar on top, put the pan in the fryer and cook at 380 degrees F for 20 minutes. Divide between plates and serve.

Nutrition: calories 273, fat 13, fiber 4, carbs 6, protein 18

Jalapeno Clouds

Prep time: 10 minutes **Cooking time:** 4 minutes
Servings: 4

Ingredients:

2 egg whites

1 jalapeno pepper

1 teaspoon almond flour

1 oz Jarlsberg cheese, grated

Directions:

Whisk the egg whites until you get the strong peaks. After this, carefully mix up egg white peaks, almond flour, and Jarlsberg cheese. Slice the jalapeno pepper on 4 slices. Preheat the air fryer to 385F. Line the air fryer basket with baking paper. With the help of the spoon make the egg white clouds on the baking paper. Top the clouds with sliced jalapeno.

Cook them for 4 minutes or until the clouds are light brown.

Nutrition: calories 75, fat 5.6, fiber 0.9, carbs 1.8, protein 5.1

Broccoli Puree

Preparation time: 5 minutes **Cooking time:** 20 minutes **Servings:** 4

Ingredients:

20 ounces broccoli florets A drizzle of olive oil

4 tablespoons basil, chopped 3 ounces butter, melted

1 garlic clove, minced

A pinch of salt and black pepper

Directions:

In a bowl, mix the broccoli with the oil, salt and pepper, toss and transfer to your air fryer's basket. Cook at 380 degrees F for 20 minutes, cool the broccoli down and put it in a blender. Add the rest of the ingredients, pulse, divide the mash between plates and serve as a side dish.

Nutrition: calories 200, fat 14, fiber 3, carbs 6, protein 7

Dill Cabbage Sauté

Preparation time: 5 minutes **Cooking time:** 20 minutes **Servings**: 4

Ingredients:

30 ounces red cabbage, shredded 4 ounces butter, melted

A pinch of salt and black pepper 1 teaspoon cinnamon powder

1 tablespoon red wine vinegar 2 tablespoons dill, chopped

Directions:

In a pan that fits your air fryer, mix the cabbage with the rest of the ingredients, toss, put the pan in the machine and cook at 390 degrees F for 20 minutes. Divide between plates and serve as a side dish.

Nutrition: calories 201, fat 17, fiber 2, carbs 5, protein 5

Coconut Celery and Broccoli Mash

Prep time: 10 minutes **Cooking time:** 5 minutes **Servings:** 2

Ingredients:

7 oz broccoli florets

1 tablespoon almond butter

½ teaspoon salt

2 oz celery stalk, chopped

2 tablespoons coconut cream

Cooking spray

Directions:

Preheat the air fryer to 400F. Then put the broccoli florets and celery stalk in the air fryer basket and spray them with cooking spray. Cook the vegetables for 5 minutes at 400F. Then put the cooked vegetables in the blender and blend them until you get a puree. After this, put the puree in the bowl. Add salt, almond butter, and coconut cream. Stir the puree with the help of the spoon.

Nutrition: calories 122, fat8.5, fiber 4.2, carbs 9.8, protein 5

Cumin Brussels Sprouts

Preparation time: 5 minutes **Cooking time:** 15 minutes **Servings**: 4

Ingredients:

1 pound Brussels sprouts, trimmed and shredded

½ cup olive oil Juice of 1 lemon

Zest of 1 lemon, grated

A pinch of salt and black pepper

¼ cup almonds, toasted and chopped

½ teaspoon cumin, crushed 1 teaspoon chili paste

Directions:

In a pan that fits the air fryer, combine the Brussels sprouts with all the other ingredients, toss, put the pan in the fryer and cook at 390 degrees F for 15 minutes. Divide between plates and serve as a side dish.

Nutrition: calories 200, fat 9, fiber 2, carbs 6, protein 9

Collard Greens with Peanuts

Prep time: 10 minutes **Cooking time:** 10 minutes **Servings:** 4

Ingredients:

2 cups collard greens, chopped

3 oz bacon, chopped

1 teaspoon butter, melted

1 oz peanuts, chopped

¼ teaspoon salt

Directions:

Preheat the air fryer to 400F. Put the bacon in the air fryer basket and cook for8 minutes. Stir it from time to time. After this, add collard greens and salt. Mix up the mixture and cook for 2 minutes more. Transfer the cooked meal in the serving plates and top with butter and peanuts.

Nutrition: calories 170, fat 13.5, fiber 1.4, carbs 2.7, protein 10.2

Parsley Zucchini Spaghetti

Preparation time: 5 minutes **Cooking time:** 15 minutes **Servings**: 4

Ingredients:

1 pound zucchinis, cut with a spiralizer

¼ cup olive oil

Salt and black pepper to the taste 6 garlic cloves, minced

½ teaspoon red pepper flakes 1 cup parmesan, grated

¼ cup parsley, chopped

Directions:

In a pan that fits your air fryer, mix all the ingredients, toss, introduce in the fryer and cook at 370 degrees F for 15 minutes. Divide between plates and serve as a side dish.

Nutrition: calories 200, fat 6, fiber 3, carbs 4, protein 5

Garlic Broccoli Rabe

Prep time: 10 minutes **Cooking time:** 20 minutes
Servings: 4

Ingredients:

7 oz broccoli rabe, roughly chopped

2 tablespoons almond flour

1 teaspoon coconut oil, melted

¼ teaspoon salt

1 tablespoon avocado oil

1 teaspoon garlic powder

Directions:

Preheat the air fryer to 355F. In the mixing bowl, mix up broccoli rabe, salt, garlic powder, and melted coconut oil. Mix up the greens and sprinkle them with almond flour. Shake them well. After this, sprinkle the broccoli rabe with avocado oil and transfer in the air fryer. Cook the greens for 20 minutes. Shake them every 5 minutes to avoid burning.

Nutrition: calories 108, fat8.6, fiber 1.7, carbs 5.5, protein 4.3

Creamy Cauliflower

Prep time: 10 minutes **Cooking time:** 25 minutes
Servings: 4

Ingredients:

8 oz cauliflower florets, boiled

½ cup ground chicken

1 tablespoon keto tomato sauce

1 tablespoon coconut oil

2 tablespoons cream cheese

½ cup Mozzarella cheese, shredded

1 teaspoon fresh parsley, chopped

1 teaspoon salt

1 teaspoon cayenne pepper

½ teaspoon basil

Directions:

Put the coconut oil in the skillet and melt it over the medium heat. Then add ground chicken, salt, cayenne pepper, and parsley. Add basil and mix up the ground chicken mixture. Cook it for 5 minutes. Then stir well and add tomato sauce. Mix up the mixture well. Put the ½ part of cauliflower florets in the air fryer pan. Then top them with ground chicken mixture.

Cover this layer with remaining cauliflower, cream cheese, and Mozzarella cheese. Cook the meal at 375F for 10 minutes.

Nutrition: calories 109, fat 7.2, fiber 1.7, carbs 4.3, protein 7.8

Goat Cheese Cauliflower and Bacon

Preparation time: 5 minutes **Cooking time:** 20 minutes **Servings**: 4

Ingredients:

8 cups cauliflower florets, roughly chopped 4 bacon strips, chopped

Salt and black pepper to the taste

½ cup spring onions, chopped 1 tablespoon garlic, minced

10 ounces goat cheese, crumbled

¼ cup soft cream cheese Cooking spray

Directions:

Grease a baking pan that fits the air fryer with the cooking spray and mix all the ingredients except the goat cheese into the pan. Sprinkle the cheese on top, introduce the pan in the machine and cook at 400 degrees F for 20 minutes. Divide between plates and serve as a side dish.

Nutrition: calories 203, fat 13, fiber 2, carbs 5, protein 9

Chinese Chili Chicken

Prep time: 15 minutes **Cooking time:** 20 minutes
Servings: 6

Ingredients:

6 chicken wings

1 tablespoon coconut aminos

1 teaspoon ground ginger

1 teaspoon salt

1 teaspoon minced garlic

2 tablespoons apple cider vinegar

1 tablespoon olive oil

1 chili pepper, chopped

Directions:

Put the chicken wings in the bowl and sprinkle with coconut aminos and ground ginger. Add salt, minced garlic, apple cider vinegar, olive oil, and chopped chili.

Mix up the chicken wings and leave them for 15 minutes to marinate. Meanwhile, preheat the air fryer to 380F. Place the marinated chicken wings in the air fryer and cook them for 20 minutes. Flip the chicken wings from time to time to avoid the burning.

Nutrition: calories 303, fat 13.2, fiber 0.1, carbs 1, protein 42.3

Cardamom and Almond Duck

Preparation time: 5 minutes **Cooking time:** 30 minutes **Servings**: 4

Ingredients:

duck legs

Juice of ½ lemon

Zest of ½ lemon, grated

tablespoon cardamom, crushed

¼ teaspoon allspice

tablespoons almonds, toasted and chopped 2 tablespoons olive oil

Directions:

In a bowl, mix the duck legs with the remaining ingredients except the almonds and toss. Put the duck legs in your air fryer's basket and cook at 380 degrees F for 15 minutes on each side. Divide the duck legs between plates, sprinkle the almonds on top and serve with a side salad.

Nutrition: calories 284, fat 12, fiber 4, carbs 6, protein 18

Duck and Strawberry Sauce

Prep time: 15 minutes **Cooking time:** 15 minutes
Servings: 4

Ingredients:

1-pound duck breast, skinless, boneless

1 tablespoon Erythritol

2 tablespoons water

1 oz strawberry

½ teaspoon salt

½ teaspoon ground paprika

¼ teaspoon ground cinnamon

1 teaspoon chili powder

1 teaspoon sesame oil

Directions:

Rub the duck breast with salt and chili powder. Then brush it with sesame oil. Preheat the air fryer to 380F.

Put the duck breast in the air fryer and cook it for 12 minutes. Meanwhile, make the sweet sauce: in the small bowl mix up Erythritol, water, ground paprika, and ground cinnamon.

Mash the strawberry and add it in the Erythritol mixture. Stir it well and microwave it for 10 seconds. Then stir the sauce and microwave it for 10 seconds more. Repeat the same steps 2 times more. Then rush the duck breast with ½ part of sweet sauce and cook for 3 minutes more. Slice the cooked duck breast and sprinkle it with remaining sauce.

Nutrition: calories 162, fat 5.8, fiber 0.5, carbs 1.2, protein 25.1

Duck with Olives

Preparation time: 5 minutes **Cooking time:** 25 minutes **Servings**: 2

Ingredients:

2 duck legs

1 teaspoon cinnamon powder 1 tablespoon olive oil

garlic clove, minced

A pinch of salt and black pepper

ounces black olives, pitted and sliced Juice of ½ lime

1 tablespoon parsley, chopped

Directions:

In a bowl, mix the duck legs with cinnamon, oil, garlic, salt and pepper, and rub well. Heat up a pan that fits the air fryer over medium-high heat, add duck legs and brown for 2-3 minutes on each side. Add the remaining ingredients to the pan, put the pan in the air fryer and cook at 400 degrees F for 10 minutes on each side. Divide between plates and serve.

Nutrition: calories 276, fat 12, fiber 4, carbs 6, protein 14

Spring Chicken Mix

Preparation time: 10 minutes **Cooking time:** 20 minutes **Servings**: 4

Ingredients:

pounds duck breast, skinless, boneless and cubed

½ cup spring onions, chopped Salt and black pepper to the taste 1 tablespoon olive oil

2 garlic cloves, minced

¼ teaspoon red pepper flakes, crushed 1 tablespoons sesame seeds, toasted

Directions:

Heat up a pan that fits your air fryer with the oil over medium heat, add the meat, toss and brown for 5 minutes. Add the rest of the ingredients except the sesame seeds, toss, introduce in the fryer and cook at 380 degrees F for 15 minutes. Add sesame seeds, toss, divide between plates and serve.

Nutrition: calories 264, fat 12, fiber 4, carbs 6, protein 17

Chicken Satay

Prep time: 10 minutes **Cooking time:** 14 minutes
Servings: 4

Ingredients:

4 chicken wings

1 teaspoon olive oil

1 teaspoon keto tomato sauce

1 teaspoon dried cilantro

½ teaspoon salt

Directions:

String the chicken wings on the wooden skewers. Then in the shallow bowl mix up olive oil, tomato sauce, dried cilantro, and salt. Spread the chicken skewers with the tomato mixture. Preheat the air fryer to 390F. Arrange the chicken satay in the air fryer and cook the meal for 10 minutes. Then flip the chicken satay on another side and cook it for 4 minutes more.

Nutrition: calories 170, fat 11.9, fiber 0.2, carbs 5.7, protein 9.8

Simple Paprika Duck

Preparation time: 5 minutes **Cooking time:** 25 minutes **Servings**: 4

Ingredients:

1 pound duck breasts, skinless, boneless and cubed Salt and black pepper to the taste

1 tablespoon olive oil

½ teaspoon sweet paprika

¼ cup chicken stock

1 teaspoon thyme, chopped

Directions:

Heat up a pan that fits your air fryer with the oil over medium heat, add the duck pieces, and brown them for 5 minutes. Add the rest of the ingredients, toss, put the pan in the machine and cook at 380 degrees F for 20 minutes. Divide between plates and serve.

Nutrition: calories 264, fat 14, fiber 4, carbs 6, protein 18

Chicken, Mushrooms and Peppers Pan

Prep time: 10 minutes **Cooking time:** 22 minutes **Servings:** 5

Ingredients:

1-pound chicken breast, skinless, boneless

1 teaspoon minced ginger

½ teaspoon minced garlic

1 tablespoon coconut aminos

1 teaspoon lemon juice

5 oz cremini mushrooms, sliced

¼ cup bell pepper, sliced

5 oz cauliflower, chopped

1 teaspoon ground paprika

½ teaspoon cayenne pepper

1 tablespoon avocado oil

1 teaspoon salt

Directions:

Preheat the air fryer to 375F. In the mixing bowl mix up sliced mushrooms, cauliflower, and bell pepper. Sprinkle the ingredients with salt, ½ tablespoon avocado oil, cayenne pepper, and ground paprika. Mix up the vegetables and place them in the air fryer basket. Cook the ingredients for 5 minutes. Then shake them well and cook for 3 minutes more. Transfer the cooked vegetables into the bowl. Then preheat the air fryer to 380F. Slice the chicken breast into the strips. Sprinkle the sliced chicken breast with minced ginger, minced garlic, and sprinkle with coconut aminos and lemon juice. Place the chicken breast in the air fryer and cook it for 13 minutes. Then add cooked vegetables and mix up the meal. Cook it for 1 minute more.

Nutrition: calories 130, fat 2.8, fiber 1.4, carbs 4.6, protein 20.7

Creamy Duck and Lemon Sauce

Preparation time: 5 minutes **Cooking time:** 25 minutes **Servings**: 4

Ingredients:

2 spring onions, chopped

2 tablespoons butter, melted 4 garlic cloves, minced

1 and ½ teaspoons coriander, ground Salt and black pepper to the taste

15 ounces tomatoes, crushed

¼ cup lemon juice

and ½ pounds duck breast, skinless, boneless and cubed

½ cup cilantro, chopped

½ cup chicken stock

½ cup heavy cream

Directions:

Heat up a pan that fits your air fryer with the butter over medium heat, add the duck pieces and cook for 5 minutes. Add the rest of the ingredients except the cilantro, toss, introduce the pan in the fryer and cook at 370 degrees F for 20 minutes. Divide between plates and serve.

Nutrition: calorie 284, fat 12, fiber 4, carbs 6, protein 17

Paprika Liver Spread

Prep time: 10 minutes **Cooking time:**8 minutes
Servings: 6

Ingredients:

1-pound chicken liver

2 tablespoons ghee

1 teaspoon salt

1 teaspoon smoked paprika

¼ cup hot water

Directions:

Preheat the air fryer to 400F. Wash and trim the chicken liver and arrange it in the air fryer basket. Cook the ingredients for 5 minutes. Then flip them on another side and cook for 3 minutes more. When the chicken liver is cooked, transfer it in the blender. Add ghee, salt, and smoked paprika. Add hot water and blend the mixture until smooth. Then transfer the cooked chicken pâté in the bowl and store it in the fridge for up to 3 days.

Nutrition: calories 167, fat 9.2, fiber 0.3, carbs 1.4, protein 18.6

www.ingramcontent.com/pod-product-compliance
Lightning Source LLC
Chambersburg PA
CBHW050220270326
41914CB00003BA/491